Table of Contents

When shopping at the grocery store, the foods you grab can greatly impact your overall health. In fact, filling your cart with a lot of refined grains, sugary drinks, and processed foods can increase inflammation and affect your health.

Therefore, filling up on healthy foods can help keep you healthy, protect against chronic diseases resistant to drugs and rid your body of toxins.

We also absorb tons of toxins every day through the air we breathe, the water we drink, the food we eat, and by just being outside in our surroundings.

So how do we get rid of these toxins that can be harmful to our body? It's through the Healing diet.

The Healing foods diet is not just a diet; It is a tool that will lead you to a total transformation of your health. This diet was designed to help everyone overcome diseases. It is designed to heal your body and improve your health by encouraging the consumption of nutritious, whole foods like fruits, veggies, legumes, healthy fats, organic meats, and healing herbs and spices.

Plus, this simple eating pattern is a great way to ensure you supply your body with a steady stream of the nutrients you need to help prevent nutritional deficiencies in your diet and to promote healthy living.

So what makes this diet unique?

This diet is unique because it involves making some simple switches in your diet compared to other complicated diets with many rules and regulations.

THE HEALING CIRRHOSIS DIET RECIPES

1. Tuna Salad

Prep: 5 mins

Total: 5 mins

Servings: 2

Ingredients

- One can of low sodium tuna
- 1 Tbs. Miracle Whip salad dressing or Karen's Faker Easy Low Sodium Mayonnaise
- 2 Tbs. Westbrae, No Sodium Mustard
- 1 boiled egg
- Green salad mix
- 1 tomato
- 1 avocado
- Fresh or dried dill weed

Directions

1. Chop the boiled egg

2. Mix with low sodium Mayonnaise, salad dressing and mustard.

3. Add other ingredients and stir

4. Place greens on plate with avocado and tomato and place ½ the tuna mix on top. That's it.

Prep: 3 mins

Cook: 15 mins

Total: 18 mins

Servings: 6

Ingredients

- 4 large potatoes, cubed (about 1-inch)
- 1/2 cup lemon juice
- 2 teaspoons mustard powder or turmeric powder
- 1/2 teaspoon cumin seeds (optional)
- 1 1/2 teaspoon sea salt
- 1 red small onion finely chopped
- 2 cloves garlic, minced
- 1/2 cup extra virgin olive oil

Directions

1. Steam the potatoes until fork tender (about 10-15 minutes).

2. In small bowl mix lemon juice, mustard or turmeric powder, cumin seeds (optional), and salt.

3. Place the steamed potatoes in a large bowl, pour the lemon juice mixture over the potatoes, add the onions and garlic and stir gently to coat the potatoes. Cover and place in the refrigerator to cool.

4. When the potatoes are cool, pour over olive oil, add fresh herbs and stir well.

5. Can be served chilled or at room temperature.

Prep: 2 mins

Total: 2 mins

Servings: 2

Ingredients

- 1/3 cup raspberries (sliced)
- 1/3 cup blueberries
- 1 cup coconut water
- 1/2 banana
- 1/3 cup low fat Greek yogurt
- 1/2 cup kale (chopped)
- 1/4 cup red beets (cooked, chopped)
- 1 tablespoon nut butter
- 1 teaspoon flax oil
- 1 scoop Further Food Collagen Peptides

Directions

1. Blend all ingredients until smooth.
2. Serve immediately.

Prep: 10 mins

Total: 10 mins

Servings: 2

Ingredients

- 1 ripe banana, peeled
- 1/2 green apple, cored and chopped
- 1 medium-sized carrot, peeled and chopped
- 1 handful baby spinach
- 1 (1/4-inch) nub turmeric root, peeled
- 1 tbsp fresh parsley, chopped
- 3 walnut halves
- 2 tbsp Hemp Protein Powder
- 1/2 lemon, juiced
- 1 pinch cinnamon, optional
- 3/4 cup unsweetened almond milk

Directions

1. Add all ingredients for the smoothie to a blender and blend until completely smooth.
2. Taste smoothie for flavor and add more cinnamon and/or some honey to taste.

5. Beets, Brocolli and Carrot soup

Prep: 15 mins

Cook: 1 hr

Total: 1 hr 15 mins

Servings: 4

Ingredients

- 3 cups water (filtered/purified)
- 1 cup organic vegetable broth
- 2 organic beets (peeled + diced)
- 2 organic carrots (sliced)
- 2 cups organic broccoli (chopped)
- 10 cloves organic garlic (freshly crushed)
- 1 organic onion (diced)
- 1/2 organic lemon (freshly squeezed)
- 2 organic bay leaves
- 1/2 teaspoon Himalayan pink salt
- 1/2 teaspoon organic ground turmeric
- 1/2 teaspoon organic dried oregano

- 1/2 teaspoon organic ground black pepper

Directions

1. Prepare the veggies:
- Slice/Dice/Cut the beets, carrots, broccoli, and onions to the size of your preference.
2. Prepare the soup:
- Add all the ingredients for the soup to a medium-size pot and bring to a boil.
- Lower the heat and simmer on low heat for approximately 1 hour, or until the veggies are soft.
- Add extra water or veggie broth if needed and adjust seasonings to your preference.

Prep: 10 mins

Cook: 10 minms

Total: 20 mins

Servings: 4

Ingredients

- One 14-ounce package extra-firm tofu
- 3 tablespoons olive oil
- 3 tablespoons crushed garlic
- Sea salt and freshly ground black pepper

Directions

1. Remove the tofu from the package and drain the water. Pat dry with paper towel and cut into 1-inch cubes.

2. Place the tofu in a large bowl with 2 tablespoons of the olive oil, the garlic and salt and pepper to taste. Mix thoroughly.

3. In a separate pan, heat the remaining tablespoon of olive oil for 1 to 2 minutes, then add the tofu mixture.

4. Sauté until the tofu is browned on all sides, 5 to 6 minutes. Serve immediately.

7. Turmeric Spiced Chickpea and Artichoke Saute

Prep: 5 mins

Cook: 7 mins

Total: 12 mins

Servings: 4

Ingredients

- 1 ½ cup cooked chickpeas (about 1 can, rinsed)
- 1 ½ cup artichoke hearts (about 1 can, rinsed)
- 3 tablespoons extra virgin olive oil
- 2 teaspoons of Superfood Turmeric
- ½ teaspoon sea salt
- ½ teaspoon cracked black pepper
- 1 tablespoon minced garlic

Directions

1. Heat a large saute pan or cast iron skillet over medium-high heat.

2. Combine chickpeas, artichoke hearts, olive oil and seasonings in a bowl to evenly coat.

3. When pan is hot, toss in all ingredients and shake pan to prevent sticking.

4. Stir mixture once a minute and cook for 5-6 minutes or until chickpeas have a nice brown crust.

5. Squeeze lemon juice over the sauté and serve immediately with whole wheat pita bread or chill for later. Mixture will hold up to three days in fridge. Enjoy!

Prep: 2 mins

Cook: 3 mins

Total: 5 mins

Servings: 1

Ingredients

- 1 cup water
- ½ cup rolled oats
- 1 tbsp chia seeds
- 2 tbsp hemp seeds
- ½ tsp cinnamon
- 1 tsp coconut sugar
- ¾ cup almond milk

Directions

1. Measure 1 cup water into a pot and bring to a boil.

2. Once the water is boiling, add oatmeal, chia and hemp seeds. Cook for 3 minutes while stirring occasionally.

3. Serve in a bowl and top with almond milk, cinnamon and coconut sugar.

9. Broccoli Salad

Prep: 5 mins

Cook: 5 mins

Total: 10 mins

Servings: 4

Ingredients

- 1 head of broccoli cut into florets and rinsed
- 1 tbsp goats butter or olive oil
- 2 tbsp heaped pomegranate seeds
- 1/2 red chilli finely sliced
- 2 handfuls nuts such as brazil nuts, finely chopped

Directions

1. Steam the broccoli until just tender, then place it in a serving bowl.
2. Add the butter or oil and mix.
3. Add the rest of the ingredients, mix and serve.

Prep: 15 mins

Total: 15 mins

Servings: 1

Ingredients

- 6 red apples
- 1 small beetroot
- 2 carrots
- 1 stalk celery
- 1/2 lemon roughly peeled
- 1 thumb length piece ginger

Directions

1. Put all the ingredients through a juicer.
2. Serve immediately

11. Sweet Potato and Carrot Soup

Prep: 10 mins

Cook: 20 mins

Total: 30 mins

Servings: 2

Ingredients

- 1/2 cup cooked lentils
- 1 sweet potato, peeled and cut in cubes
- 3 carrots, peeled and roughly chopped
- 1 parsnip, peeled and roughly chopped
- 1 onion, peeled and cut in quarters
- 3 garlic cloves, crushed
- 1 teaspoon turmeric powder
- 1 teaspoon cumin powder
- 1/4 teaspoon sea salt
- 2 cups low sodium vegetable broth, warm
- 1 teaspoon grated ginger
- 1 pinch chili powder

- 1 teaspoon coconut oil
- fresh parsley, flaxseed, toasted mixed nuts, coconut milk - to garnish

Directions

1. Heat the oven at 165°C/329°F.
2. Line a baking sheet with baking paper, add the sweet potato, carrots, parsnip, onion, garlic, turmeric, cumin, chili, coconut oil, salt and toss to combine.
3. Roast for 20 minutes, then transfer into the blender.
4. Add the warm broth, grated ginger and cooked lentil and process to obtain a smooth cream
5. Serve warm, garnished with mixed nuts and seeds, parsley and coconut milk.

Prep: 10 mins

Cook: 20 mins

Total: 30 mins

Servings: 2

Ingredients

- Pasta (whole-grain or gluten-free)
- 1 cup No-salt canned cannellini beans
- 2 cups No-salt canned diced tomatoes
- 1 1/2 cups Frozen vegetables - Italian blend
- 2 cups Kalamata olives
- 1/4 cup Italian seasoning blend
- 1 tsp Garlic powder
- 2 pinches

Directions

1. Cook the whole grain pasta according to directions on the package.

2. Drain and rinse the cannellini beans. In a pot over medium heat, combine the beans, diced tomatoes (no need to drain them), frozen vegetables, olives, italian seasoning, and garlic powder.

3. Heat until warm throughout. Serve over the cooked pasta.

13. Whole-Wheat Spaghetti with Lemon, Basil, and Salmon

Prep: 10 mins

Cook: 10 mins

Total: 20 mins

Servings: 4

Ingredients

- 1/2 pound whole grain or whole wheat spaghetti
- 1 clove garlic, minced
- 2 tablespoons extra-virgin olive oil
- 1/2 teaspoon salt, plus more for seasoning
- 1/2 teaspoon freshly ground black pepper, plus more for seasoning
- 1 tablespoon olive oil
- 4 (4-ounce) pieces wild caught, Alaskan salmon
- 1/4 cup chopped fresh basil leaves
- 3 tablespoons capers
- 1 lemon, zested
- 2 tablespoons lemon juice

- 2 cups fresh organic baby spinach leaves

Directions

1. Cook pasta as directed on package until al dente (about 8-10 minutes).
2. When the pasta is finished cooking, drain it and toss the pasta in a large bowl together the garlic, extra-virgin olive oil, salt, and pepper. Set aside.
3. Warm the olive oil in a medium skillet over medium-high heat. Season the salmon with salt and pepper. Add the fish to the pan and cook until medium-rare (or to your liking), about 2 minutes per side, depending on the thickness of the fish. Remove the salmon from the pan.
4. Add the basil, capers, lemon zest, and lemon juice to the spaghetti mixture and toss to combine. Set out 4 serving plates or shallow bowls. Place 1/2 cup spinach in each bowl. Top with 1/4 of the pasta. Top each mound of pasta with a piece of salmon. Serve immediately.

Prep: 10 mins

Cook: 10 mins

Total: 20 mins

Servings: 6

Ingredients

- 12 ounces fettuccini, uncooked
- 1 tablespoon olive oil
- 2 tablespoons unsalted butter
- 2 garlic cloves
- 3/4 cup red bell pepper
- 2 tablespoons all-purpose flour
- 1/3 cup white wine
- 1 cup low-sodium chicken broth
- 1/2 cup half and half creamer
- 2 teaspoons dried parsley flakes
- 1/4 teaspoon black pepper
- 1/4 cup grated Parmesan cheese

Directions

1. Mince garlic and slice red bell pepper.

2. Cook fettuccini according to package directions, omitting the salt. Drain and set aside.

3. In a medium saucepan melt butter and combine with the olive oil. Add garlic and red bell pepper. Sauté 1 to 2 minutes until vegetables are soft.

4. Slowly stir flour into the pan. Cook 1 minute until smooth.

5. Add wine gradually, stirring until smooth.

6. Add broth, creamer, parsley and black pepper. Stir to blend.

7. Gradually add Parmesan cheese. Reduce heat to low and cook 5 to 7 minutes until mixture starts to simmer. Stir occasionally.

8. Toss the sauce with the drained fettuccini.

Prep: 5 mins

Cook: 40 mins

Total: 45 mins

Servings: 5

Ingredients

- 300 g bacon lardons
- 1 leek, sliced
- 1 carrot, diced
- 1 celery stick, sliced
- 1 onion, chopped
- 2 1/2 pints vegetable stock
- 400 g chopped tomatoes
- 1 cans cannellini or butter beans
- 50 g small pasta e.g. macaroni
- 1 handful basil leaves, torn
- 1 savoy cabbage, shredded

Directions

1. Start by heating some olive oil in a large, lidded pan. Add the bacon, leek, carrot, celery, and onion. Simmer gently for 8min.

2. Add the stock and tomatoes. Cover and leave to simmer for 20min. Resist the temptation to pour yourself a glass of wine.

3. Throw in the beans and pasta. Leave them to cook for 10min.

4. Add the basil and cabbage to the top of the soup so they can lightly steam. When they're cooked, but still have crunch, serve up a bowl and save the rest to eat in the week.

Prep: 15 mins

Cook: 3 hrs

Total: 3 hrs 15 mins

Servings: 6

Ingredients

- 2 medium onions chopped
- 1 teaspoon olive oil or non-stick spray
- 2 cloves garlic minced
- 32 ounces tomatoes, canned, no salt added
- 12 ounces tomato paste no salt added
- 1 cup red wine
- 1 cup water
- 2 teaspoons oregano dried
- 1 teaspoon black pepper
- 1 teaspoon sugar

Directions

1. In a deep saucepan, cook onion in oil or non-stick spray until soft.
2. Add remaining ingredients and simmer for 2 to 3 hours.
3. Taste after 1½ hours and adjust seasoning.
4. Sauteed mushrooms are a great addition.

Prep: 20 mins

Cook: 10 mins

Total: 30 mins

Servings: 6

Ingredients

- 2 ½ cups uncooked pasta, preferably whole-wheat (6.8 ounces)
- 4 cups chopped raw broccoli
- 2 large boneless, skinless chicken breasts cut into bite-sized cubes (1 pound)
- ¼ cup plus 1 tablespoon all-purpose flour
- ¼ teaspoon coarse kosher salt
- ¼ teaspoon ground pepper or to taste
- 2 teaspoons extra-virgin olive oil, divided
- 3 cloves garlic, minced
- 1 cup reduced-sodium chicken broth
- 2/3 cup non-fat or low-fat milk

- ¼ cup half-and-half

- 1 ½ teaspoon Dijon mustard

- 1 teaspoon chopped thyme

- 1 cup grated Parmesan cheese plus more for serving.

Directions

1. Bring a large pot of water to a boil over high heat. Cook pasta 3 minutes less than time according to package instructions. Add broccoli and continue cooking for the remaining 3 minutes. Drain and keep warm.

2. Meanwhile, toss chicken with flour, salt and pepper in a medium bowl. Heat 2 teaspoons oil in a large non-stick skillet over medium-high heat. Add the chicken, leaving excess flour in the bowl. Cook chicken, stirring occasionally, until browned on one or two sides, about 4 minutes. Remove to a plate and keep warm (it will continue cooking in step 4).

3. Wipe out skillet with a clean paper towel. Reduce heat to medium.

4. Heat the remaining 2 teaspoons oil in the skillet. Add garlic, and cook stirring until fragrant, 30 to 90 seconds. Stir in the chicken and any juice from the plate.

5. Dust on the remaining flour from the bowl, and stir to combine. Add broth and stir until the flour is incorporated. Increase heat to high and bring to a simmer stirring often. Stir in milk, half and half, Dijon and thyme, reduce heat to medium and return to a simmer, stirring. Simmer, stirring occasionally until the chicken is cooked through and the sauce is thick, about 4 minutes. Remove from heat and add 1 cup Parmesan. Stir until the sauce is smooth. Add pasta and broccoli, and stir until combined. Serve topped with additional Parmesan.

18. Quick Veggie Buckwheat Noodle Bowl

Prep: 5 mins

Cook: 15 mins

Total: 20 mins

Servings: 1

Ingredients

- 2 ounces (1 ¼ cup cooked) organic soba noodles (or other whole wheat noodle)
- ¾ cup broccolini stems (sliced lengthwise)
- ¾ cup green cabbage or bok choy (chopped into ribbons)
- 2 teaspoons toasted sesame oil
- 2 cups vegetable, chicken or mushroom broth
- ½ teaspoon Chinese 5-spice
- 2 small French breakfast or globe radishes (sliced into coins)
- 1 small jalapeno (seeded and sliced into coins)

Directions

1. Cook noodles about a minute less than the package suggests, drain and toss with 1 teaspoon of sesame oil to prevent sticking.
2. Steam broccolini and cabbage (in same vessel is fine) for no more than 1 minute.
3. Heat a medium skillet over a medium-high flame and add the remaining 1 teaspoon of sesame oil
4. Sauté broccolini and cabbage in the skillet for about 5 minutes or until just lightly charred. Remove from heat and set aside.
5. Bring broth to a boil, stir in 5 spice and noodles and remove from heat.
6. Pour broth, noodles, and vegetables into one bowl
7. Top with chilled radish and jalapeno. Serve.

19. Low Sodium Hungarian Goulash

Prep: 10 mins

Cook: 1 hr

Total: 1 hr 10 mins

Servings: 6

Ingredients

- Lean stew meat
- Sweet paprika (this is the secret ingredient)
- A little garlic powder or 1 crushed clove
- 1 can diced tomatoes
- 1 can tomato sauce
- ½ onion chopped.
- Pasta

Directions

1. Cut the meat into smaller pieces, cover them with Sweet Paprika, and brown them in a couple of tablespoons of olive oil.

2. After taking the meat out, toss it in the onion and garlic with a little more olive oil and let them sauté for about 10 minutes on low.

3. Pour it all in a pot on the stove and add the tomatoes. Cover it and cook on medium.

4. After about an hour of simmering on low, you can add to some shell macaroni or use any type of pasta.

Prep: 10 mins

Cook: 20 mins

Total: 30 mins

Servings: 2

Ingredients

- 1/2 package (about 6 ounces) of your favorite pasta.
- 3-4 tablespoons of olive oil - or any tasty vegetable oil.
- 1 tablespoon of chopped or crushed garlic - fresh or from the jar.
- 1 teaspoon of dried red chile pepper flakes.
- 2 tablespoons of dried or fresh grated parmesan cheese - optional.

(If you have any fresh herbs on hand, add a chopped teaspoon for extra flavor).

Directions

1. Start your pasta boiling, and cook according to package directions.
2. First add crushed garlic to an unheated medium size pan (but large enough to add cooked pasta). Don't add garlic from the jar to a hot pan or it will splatter and make a mess.
3. Next add oil and turn on the heat to medium/low. Saute garlic for 3- 5 minutes until it starts to lightly brown. Watch garlic closely as it is easy to burn. Add red chile flakes and mix well.
4. Pasta should be done by now (okay to precook pasta). Mix in pasta - heat through. Finally, sprinkle on dried parmesan cheese (or fresh grated) and any fresh herbs you may have on hand (optional). Enjoy.

Prep: 20 mins

Cook: 30 mins

Total: 50 mins

Servings: 10

Ingredients

- 4 cups dry whole wheat fusilli (can use penne pasta or similar)
- 1 small onion, finely chopped
- 2 (6 ounce) cans solid white tuna, water packed, well drained (can use 3 cans)
- 2 (10 ounce) cans fat free cream of celery soup or (10 ounce) cans cream of mushroom soup, undiluted
- ½ cup low-fat mayonnaise
- 1 cup skim milk or 1 cup 1% low-fat milk
- 1 (10 ounce) can sliced mushrooms, well drained
- 1 tablespoon Mrs. Dash seasoning mix

- ½ teaspoon garlic powder

- ½ teaspoon coarse black pepper (or to taste)

- 1 cup grated reduced-fat cheddar cheese (or to taste)

Directions

1. Set oven to 350 degrees F.
2. Grease an 11 x 7 or 13 x 9-inch baking dish with cooking spray (or use a casserole dish large enough to hold the mixture).
3. Boil the pasta in a large pot of boiling water, drain then transfer to a large bowl.
4. Add in onion and tuna; toss to combine.
5. In a saucepan heat soup with milk until smooth.
6. Stir in mushrooms mayonnaise, Mrs Dash seasoning, garlic powder and black pepper until combined; pour into the bowl and toss to combine.
7. Transfer mixture to prepared baking dish.
8. Bake for about 30 minutes.

9. Remove from oven then sprinkle with cheddar cheese, return to oven for 2-4 minutes to melt the cheese.

Prep: 10 mins

Cook: 20 mins

Total: 30 mins

Servings: 6

Ingredients

- 1 1/2 teaspoons kosher salt
- 1 teaspoon fresh ground black pepper
- 1/2 teaspoon garlic powder
- 2 pounds boneless chicken thighs, trimmed
- 2 tablespoons olive oil
- 6 cloves garlic, smashed or coarsely chopped
- 1 cup chicken broth
- 1/2 cup heavy cream
- 1/4 cup mascarpone cheese
- 1 1/2 tablespoons flour
- 1/2 teaspoon crushed red pepper flakes
- 2 tablespoons fresh chopped parsley to garnish

Directions

1. In a small bowl mix together the salt, pepper and garlic powder. Sprinkle the mixture on the chicken thighs.
2. Heat olive oil in a large skillet over medium-high heat. Place the chicken evenly into the skillet and cook until browned on each side, 4-5 minutes per side.
3. While the chicken is cooking, whisk together the broth, cream, mascarpone, flour, and red pepper flakes.
4. When the chicken is browned, add in the garlic and cook for 1 minute while stirring.
5. Reduce the heat to medium-low. Pour in the broth mixture, stir to combine and cook for 10 minutes, until the mixture has thickened, stirring occasionally.
6. Sprinkle with fresh parsley, and serve warm.

23. Chicken and Black Bean Salad

Prep: 10 mins

Total: 10 mins

Servings: 4

Ingredients

- 8 oz chicken breasts (cooked and shredded such as rotisserie)
- 8 c lettuce or mixed greens of choice
- 1 c cucumber (thinly sliced)
- 2 tomatoes (diced)
- 1 c black beans (drained and rinsed)
- 1 clove garlic (grated)
- ¼ c scallions (diced)
- ¼ c cilantro (chopped)
- 1 tsp cumin
- 1 Juice and zest of lime
- 2 tbs extra virgin olive oil
- Salt and pepper to taste

Directions

1. In a large salad bowl, combine chicken with lettuce, cucumber, tomatoes and black beans.
2. In a small bowl, whisk together garlic, scallions, cilantro, cumin, lime juice/zest.
3. Slowly drizzle in the olive oil and whisk to emulsify.
4. Pour dressing over the salad and season with salt/pepper to taste.

Prep: 5 mins

Cook: 30 mins

Total: 35 mins

Servings: 4

Ingredients

- 4 cups Chicken Bone Broth
- 2 Smart Chicken boneless, skinless chicken breasts
- 14 ounces chickpeas (drained and rinsed)
- ¼ cup lemon juice
- salt and pepper (to taste)
- 1 cup cooked bulgur wheat
- minced parsley (optional garnish)

Directions

1. Heat the Smart Chicken Classic Chicken Bone Broth in a large soup pot over medium-high heat. Bring to a boil then add the chicken breasts. Boil

the chicken breasts until tender, about 12-14 minutes. Remove chicken from the pot and set aside.

2. Stir in the chickpeas and lemon juice plus a pinch of salt and pepper then reduce heat to low and simmer.

3. Shred the chicken or roughly chop it before returning to the pot. Check for seasoning and adjust accordingly. Return heat to high to warm through.

4. Divide the cooked bulgur wheat between four soup bowls then ladle each with chicken and chickpea soup mixture. Garnish with minced parsley to serve.

25. Apple Almond Galette

Prep: 45 mins

Cook: 45 mins

Total: 1 hr 30 mins

Servings: 2

Ingredients

- 4 baking apples, peeled, cored and sliced thin
- 1 tablespoon butter
- 2 teaspoons ground cinnamon
- ⅛ teaspoon ground ginger
- 2 tablespoons brown sugar
- 9 individual Stevia packets
- 2 teaspoons almond extract
- 1 store-bought 9" layer pie crust

Directions

1. Over medium low heat, cook butter, apples, cinnamon, ginger and brown sugar for 5 to 10 minutes; until the apples become soft.

2. Turn off the heat and stir in the Stevia and the almond extract.

3. Pre–heat your oven to 400 degree F.

4. Roll out the pie crust onto a cookie sheet.

5. Pour the apple mixture into the middle of the pie crust.

6. Fold the pie crust over the apples about 3", leaving the center uncovered.

7. Pinch the creases together and bake for 30 minutes or until the pie crust is golden brown.

26. Microwave High Protein Rice

Prep: 10 mins

Cook: 10 mins

Total: 20 mins

Servings: 2

Ingredients

- 6 tablespoons unsalted butter
- 2 cups marshmallow crème
- 1 cup whey protein powder
- 5 cups rice crispy cereal

Directions

1. In a large bowl, melt butter in microwave for 1 minute.
2. Add marshmallow crème and microwave for 30 seconds; stir. Microwave 30 seconds more and stir until well blended.

3. Quickly add protein powder and mix until smooth.

4. Quickly add pre-measured rice crispy cereal and mix until coated.

5. Pour into a greased 13" x 9" pan and press down evenly.

6. Cool, and then cut into 12 bars, 3" x 4" each.

Prep: 20 mins

Cook: 50 mins

Total: 1 hr 10 mins

Servings: 2

Ingredients

- 5 Granny Smith Apples, peeled, cored and sliced
- ¼ cup lemon juice
- ¼ cup Caramel Flavoring, sugar free
- ⅓ cup All Purpose (AP) flour
- ¼ cup butter
- 1 cup Oatmeal
- 2 Tablespoons cinnamon
- Butter spray

Directions

1. Toss sliced apples in lemon juice; pour off any extra lemon juice.

2. Soak apple slices in caramel flavoring for 10 minutes.

3. Pre-heat oven to 375 degrees Fahrenheit.

4. Lightly oil an 8X8 pan, place apples in the bottom.

5. In a bowl mix flour, oatmeal and cinnamon together; then cut in the butter, until you have small pieces, sprinkle the mixture over the top of the apples.

6. Bake for 40 minutes; spray the top with a butter spray and bake for another 5 minutes.

Prep: 45 mins

Cook: 1 hr

Total: 1 hr 45 mins

Servings: 2

Ingredients

- 2 cups Red Seedless Grapes, each grape sliced in half
- 1⅓ cups Walnut Halves, chopped into small pea-size pieces
- 1¼ cups Pomegranate Infused Ocean Spray Dried Cranberries, 1- 6-ounce package
- 4 stalks Celery, chopped into quarter-inch pieces
- 7 medium-sized Gala Apples skin on
- 8 fluid ounce bottle of Maple Grove Farms of Vermont Fat-Free Cranberry Balsamic Dressing

Directions

1. Rinse cluster of red grapes and separate from the stem. Use paring knife and slice each grape in half. Place sliced grapes in extra large mixing bowl.

2. Measure walnut halves into measuring cup. Can use a nut chopper to chop nuts into pea size pieces or put walnuts in a plastic sandwich baggie, seal and use the bottom of the 1 cup measure to gently press on the walnuts to break the walnuts into pea size like pieces. Add chopped nuts to the extra large mixing bowl with the slice red grapes.

3. Add one 6 ounce bag of dried pomegranate infused cranberries to the grape and walnut mixture.

4. Rinse, clean and chop celery in quarter inch pieces, add to the grape, walnut, and dried cranberry mixture.

5. Rinse the seven Gala apples, slice in half vertically and core the apples. Make 5 apple wedges and then slice the wedges into bite size, quarter in

pieces. Add chopped apple pieces to the rest of the mixture.

6. Pour the 8 fluid ounce bottle of cranberry dressing over the entire mixture. Stir the ingredients making sure that the dressing is incorporated and covers all of the ingredients. Chill and serve.

Prep: 40 mins

Cook: 30 mins

Total: 1 hr 10 mins

Servings: 3

Ingredients

- 1 teaspoon Canola oil
- 1 large yellow onion, diced
- 4 stalks of celery, diced
- 2 Granny Smith apples, peeled, cored and diced
- 2 tablespoons ground sage
- 1 tablespoon poultry spice
- 1½ cups apple cider
- 1 cup low–sodium chicken stock
- 12 cups of cubed low–sodium bread (¾ to 1 whole loaf)

Directions

1. In a large fry pan, add oil, onions, celery and apples and sauté until onions are translucent.
2. Add sage, poultry spice, apple cider and chicken stock; simmer for 10 minutes.
3. Place cubed bread on a cooking sheet and bake in a pre-heated 400 degree F oven until the bread is brown, turning the cubes occasional to brown all sides.
4. When bread cubes are brown add to the fry pan and mix together.
5. Bake the dressing in a covered 9 X 13 pan in a 350° F oven for 20 to 30 minutes.

Prep: 10 mins

Cook: 10 mins

Total: 20 mins

Servings: 2

Ingredients

- 4 whole eggs
- 1 cup cauliflower
- 3 cups fresh spinach
- 1 garlic clove minced
- 1/4 cup bell pepper chopped
- 1/4 cup onion chopped
- 1/4 teaspoon black pepper
- 1 tablespoon oil of choice coconut or avocado oil is good for high heat
- fresh parsley and spring onion for garnish
- *optional tomatoes on side if no potassium restriction

Directions

1. Beat eggs with pepper until light and fluffy, set aside.
2. Heat oil over medium heat in large skillet.
3. Add onions and peppers to skillet and sauté until peppers are translucent and golden.
4. Add garlic, stirring quickly to combine and immediately adding cauliflower and spinach.
5. Sauté vegetables, turn heat to medium-low and cover for 5 minutes.
6. Add eggs, stirring to combine with vegetables.
7. When the eggs are cooked thoroughly, top with fresh parsley or spring onions (If no potassium restriction feel free to serve with a side of bright fresh tomatoes topped with cracker black pepper). A touch of feta or a strong sharp cheese would also be delicious with these.